THE ROCK CARLING FELLOWSHIP

1987

# The Patient's Dilemma

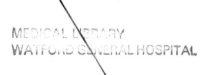

THE ROCK CARLING FELLOWSHIP

1987

# THE PATIENT'S DILEMMA

## Sir Cecil Clothier
KCB, QC

*Chairman, Police Complaints Authority*
*Formerly the Parliamentary Commissioner*
*and Health Service Commissioner*

## THE NUFFIELD PROVINCIAL HOSPITALS TRUST

Published by the
Nuffield Provincial Hospitals Trust
3 Prince Albert Road, London NW1 7SP
ISBN 0 900574 68 2
©Nuffield Provincial Hospitals Trust, 1988

Designed by Bernard Crossland
PRINTED IN GREAT BRITAIN BY
BURGESS & SON (ABINGDON) LTD
ABINGDON OXFORDSHIRE

# THE AUTHOR

Sir Cecil Clothier was born in 1919 and after seven years of service in the Royal Signals during the Second World War, began to practice at the Bar and was appointed Queen's Counsel in 1965. Thereafter his practice developed in medico-legal topics and in 1972 he was appointed by Sir Keith Joseph to conduct an inquiry into the death of six patients within a few hours, resulting from contaminated infusion fluid. Later in that year he was appointed a legal assessor to the General Medical and General Dental Council. He served on the Merrison Committee on the regulation of the medical profession and from 1976 to 1978 was a member of the Royal Commission on the National Health Service. Contemporaneously with these activities, Sir Cecil was in practice at the Bar (with a special interest in adverse drug reactions) and as a part-time judge until 1978, when he was appointed Parliamentary Commissioner for Administration and Health Service Commissioner. After six years in those posts he was appointed Chairman of the Police Complaints Authority. He was made a Knight Commander of the Bath in 1982 and an Honorary Fellow of Lincoln College, Oxford in 1984. He is also an Honorary Member of the Association of Anaesthetists of Great Britain and Ireland.

# CONTENTS

# PREFACE

When I was invited to write this modest treatise I was alarmed by the extreme distinction of my predecessors. Each was deeply learned in some field of medicine. Those of their Rock Carling monographs which I read confirmed my belief that each had studied the chosen topic profoundly. I could claim no fraction of their achievements in scholarship or practice. But I have a profession of my own in which I achieved, over nearly thirty years, a reasonable competence. It is a profession which develops to pathological proportions the critical faculty. To the advocate there is no such thing as the proposition or axiom, the belief or the motive, which cannot be turned over and over in the search for flaws. Like the American doctor's definition of a healthy person as one who has not been sufficiently studied, so to the advocate every proposition, examined for long enough, turns out to have a tiny weakness in it. Perhaps, I thought, the application of the critical faculty of the advocate to the delivery of health care (but with less fervour perhaps than is induced by a well-marked brief) might yield a few strands of thought hitherto unnoticed.

Then again, I recalled from my own life in practice how often I had learned from untutored men and women things about my own behaviour as an advocate and about the principles which I held to be unassailable, which came to me as a shock. I recalled how often I had gone home at the end of a day in court with the penetrating comment of a witness, who might have been a doctor but was just as likely to be an artisan, rankling in my mind still. The comment rankled because I knew it to be an accurate and a just criticism by a lay intelligence from which I would do well to learn. I hope that I did. I certainly remember some of the lessons to this day.

However, this is a very modest contribution to an important and continuing appraisal of the medical profession as practised in this country. 'He has much to be modest about', I almost hear someone say, in the sour witticism which must first have been coined by a lawyer. But recalling the modesty of most of those persons who were in effect my 'patients' and of how much I learned from them, I offer this slight work, no more than a collection of essays, in the hope that it may perhaps set trains of thought running in more learned minds in the field of medicine.

# ACKNOWLEDGMENTS

I acknowledge with gratitude the kindness of a friend deeply versed in the ways of the National Health Service who read a draft of this monograph and made numerous invaluable suggestions for its improvement.

I am also greatly indebted to Mrs Gillian McWalter who with unfailing patience typed a dozen versions of this monograph from my manuscripts.

# Introduction

'My dear friends, I come to complayne upon you—
but to yourselves.'
THOMAS CAREW 1598–1639

One sometimes hears a person say: 'I have never had a day's illness in my life!' My first reaction to this extraordinary statement is to wonder if it can possibly be true and if so, whether a life has been properly lived which has included no share in the sufferings inseparable for most people from living. An excessive stoicism about life's ups and downs seems neither desirable nor particularly praiseworthy. Most people complain a good deal about those departures from complete health or comfort which afflict everyone from time to time. We tell each other of extremes of heat, cold, or rain, of headaches and influenza: and we expect these recitals of far from extraordinary facts to be listened to. Occasionally we have something more majestic to relate—an admission to hospital, an operation, or an unpleasant accident. It is a sacred human duty to listen to all this and if possible actually to be moved by it. Obviously this is easier when the subject is closer by reason of family or friendship. It is harder when no previous acquaintance exists by which to establish the duty of attention.

One definition of complaint in the *Oxford English Dictionary* is: 'The expression of suffering passing into that of grievance and blame.' This is an interesting sequence, suggesting that tolerance of a limited degree of suffering, not in silence, is to be expected of the reasonable person, but that there comes a point at which continued or aggravated suffering is a legitimate cause for protest. Finally, extended suffering seems to call for the allocation of blame, to the gods, to other people

I

or sometimes to the sufferer himself. It is interesting, too, that the same noun serves to indicate both the expression of suffering and the symptom causing it. Thus one may say: 'He suffers from a distressing but common complaint.' This merging of the physical disorder with the expression of it suggests that to speak out about grief and suffering is natural and expected, while an excessive stoicism is neither. There is a kind of catharsis in complaining, just as it seems now to be established that grieving after bereavement is necessary to the recovery of good mental health. It is upon these grounds that I proposed above a social duty to listen to complaints, whether of ill-health or any other legitimate ground of grievance. The relationship between doctor or nurse and patient is a professionally acquired and special form of this duty.

Although skilled and effective treatment of illness is obviously of the greatest importance, I suggest that the first essential in the delivery of good health care is to listen to the complaint of the patient, however tiresome or irrelevant that may seem, when it is possible to do so. 'He will eventually', a wise doctor said, 'tell you what is the matter with him.' Listening is not so usually or so easily done as it might seem. The increasing use of diagnostic equipment of great sophistication and accuracy, together with the increasing pressure on the time of doctors in the Health Service, tempts them to curtail the patient's recitals and get him on his way round the diagnostic departments. But if complaining is a natural form of therapy, it remains so despite the acquisition of ingenious diagnostic aids which may more certainly and specifically confirm the diagnosis: and it may be a therapy which conditions the patient to be receptive to the more positive therapeutic measures which the doctor will later recommend. The old army maxim: 'Time spent in reconnaissance is seldom wasted' may here be in point. Listening to the patient is like gazing at the terrain over which it is proposed to move, looking for unusual features which may not immediately strike the eye.

## Introduction

The burden of this short treatise is the close relationship between doctor or nurse and patient and the way in which each perceives the delivery and the receipt of medical care from their respective standpoint. My authorities for the propositions I later advance are therefore the repeated complaints and the responses to them which I had to investigate as Health Service Commissioner for six years. Save in the periodic reports issued by that Office, dull reading indeed, these sources of grievance are not documented. It follows that my work is not heavily annotated with bibliographic footnotes, as are the works of those who study the Health Service as an entity, about which much has been written.

I have tried to avoid entrenching upon clinical ground, although on occasion I have unavoidably come rather close to the borderline, but then only to point out how certain kinds of treatment appear to the patient. An example is the extent to which sedation is sometimes thought necessary, which I have questioned with I hope becoming diffidence, in some thoughts on Intensive Therapy Units (ITUs).

I have not dealt at all with the large and important sphere of delivery of health care in general practice. The source material available to me in that area is largely anecdotal, because complaints about general practitioners were and still are outside the jurisdiction of the Health Service Commissioner: whereas the volume of recorded complaint from the hospital service is such as to afford a basis from which to draw reasonable inferences.

Some may think that what I have written is much coloured by personal experience. It is true that I have been a patient in hospital and that on a fairly considerable scale. I think that that might be a pre-requisite of writing a monograph on this topic. But I was singularly fortunate in finding myself on each occasion in some of the best hospitals in the country, all in the National Health Service, where the delivery of care was so good that it would be difficult to find a ground of complaint of

3

any kind. If any of them remember me as a patient and read this treatise, I hope that they will realise that I use my experiences in their care only as a standard of excellence against which to measure the performance of others. It is regrettably one of the features of an organization as large as the National Health Service that disparities in performance can be quite wide, as between one hospital and another and even one Region and another. It may be that this is an inevitable consequence of the differing capacities of human beings, so irritating to planners. But in medicine as in industry, politics, sport, or any other human activity one cares to think of, there are those who excel and those who return a steady and valuable performance. It is probable that each category is necessary to the existence of the other. Those who propose the abolition of excellence on the ground that it implies inequality (and I have heard so abominable a doctrine propounded quite seriously at a significant level) are fighting against an instinct to excel which is as powerful as the instinct for survival of the species. It is a contest which they are bound to lose, therefore, and we must be grateful for that. But the concomitant is that some hospitals deliver medical care which may be intrinsically identical with the best, yet which appears less so for lack of skill or care in the process of delivery. It is to that aspect of inequality that I address much of what follows. It is not enough in human affairs merely to do a competent or even an excellent piece of professional work. It is necessary also to make that appear to be the case. Hence the now weary aphorism that justice must not only be done but be seen to be done.

Finally by way of introduction I must apologize for and explain my decision after much thought to refer quite often to the patient as 'he'. This is not merely because as between the sexes, the male is much the more likely to complain about very little in the way of discomfort (that euphemism for considerable agony so beloved of the profession) or inconvenience, although I believe that to be true.[1] It is because I find it wearisome to read an article or other publication which conscientiously refers at every turn to 'he or she' and 'him or her' so as to make the point that women are not left out. The construction soon becomes cumbersome and irritating and I hope that my female readers will accept that I refer to patient-man as one refers to Neanderthal man, in a purely generic and not very flattering sense.

1. See Marplan opinion poll for NAHA, 1987, wherein 80 per cent of females thought well of the NHS, as against 72 per cent of males.

# 1
# A Special Relationship

'Fate chooses your relations ...'
ABBÉ DELILLE, *Malheur et Pitié*

A common greeting among the Greeks is: 'Health to you'. In this country we are disposed to say: 'How do you do?' on first meeting and: 'How are you?' on renewing an acquaintance. Nowadays we seldom expect an answer to the first question, but the second question usually evokes a reply, although the candour of it will depend upon the closeness of the acquaintance. Yet those conventional and often unthinking phrases recognize that the most important concern we can have for another human being is about his or her health: and of all the personal relationships we can engage in, that of caring for the sick is the closest and most demanding.

The formation of a relationship between two human beings is one of the most subtle and mysterious aspects of human behaviour. One may pass by a thousand people in the street without expressing or feeling the slightest concern about them, because nothing links us to them directly. Nor does the law recognize any positive duty of care owed by one being to another until the crucial link is somehow formed. One may stand on a seashore and see a man struggling for life a quarter of a mile out to sea; one may say to oneself: 'I am not a strong swimmer, just a length or two of the local pool. I am married to a woman I love and I have two young children. If I try to help that man I may lose strength, drown and leave my family to struggle on alone. I will not therefore try to help him.' There is no legal wrong in such a decision, nor should there be any sense of moral failure, although most would recall such an experience with unhappiness ever afterwards.

6

## A Special Relationship

But as soon as a particular bond is formed between two beings, the duty of care springs, unseen and unheard, into an existence both powerful and permanent. The bond may be formed in many ways, ranging from the obvious ties of love and family affection to the sharing of terrible experiences. But the bond most surely springs into being when one person submits himself to the clinical care of doctor and nurse. What is more, the law recognizes, as it does when two persons marry, that a duty of care is now owed by one to the other, so that failure in the fulfilment of that duty may be publicly recognized and reprehended by a court of law.

Because the balance of activity in the relationship lies with doctor and nurse while the patient's role is largely passive, there is little that a patient can do which calls for recognition of a legal duty to do it. For my part, I believe that patients, while untroubled by a concept of legal duty, should recognize a moral duty towards those who care for them. Nor is it particularly difficult to define such a duty. To start with, it would certainly include being patient. It would embrace also the proper expression of gratitude from time to time, evenness of temper, acceptance of the regime, and a conscious effort to get better. No doubt there are other aspects as well. These obligations may be difficult for the sick to achieve, perhaps by reason of the very illnesses from which they suffer.

\*       \*       \*

Illness takes many forms and I am not writing of those minor indispositions for which self-care and a little homely sympathy are appropriate. Rather I am thinking of that degree of malady which brings about surrender. For surrender it is when illness is of that degree which forces us to abandon the attempt to cure ourselves and to submit to the care and skill of others. That submission will sooner or later require us to lie down and acquiesce in the attentions to our bodies of those who are still vertical. This is a most important difference between the well

7

and the ill. The verticality of mankind is in any case recently acquired, precarious, and easily disturbed, and the fallen are at a terrible disadvantage with respect to the upright. In the field of strife or battle it is vital to remain erect. Deliberately to abandon that posture, on someone's order and while conscious, is an act of submission.

The distinction between the comparatively vanquished and their gentle captors remains even when the patient is up and about. The observant patient will note the glance of the hospital staff or visitor towards his wrist to detect whether he is to be numbered among the upright or the fallen. If the telltale bond is seen, the special look of kindly sympathy and compassion is immediately assumed and easily recognized, whereas the healthy stranger receives no second glance.

Defeat does not come easily to some. Nor for that matter does victory. For some their pride is such that surrender holds only bitterness: and for others victory holds only triumph. Neither group will be able to sustain the loving relationship which can give joy to doctor, nurse, and patient in equal measure.

The best delivery of health care will pass from one to the other of two people having the temperament to give and to receive with equal grace: for kind and appreciative receiving is as important as warm and generous giving. If the delivery of health care does not satisfy the patient, it is as likely to be the fault of the patient as of the doctor or nurse. Proverbs are supposed to encapsulate received truths: for my part I find them for the most part untrue or immoral or both. None is more pernicious than that which says: 'It take two to make a quarrel'. Plainly it takes only one quarrelsome person.

It remains however the fact that some doctors and nurses possess in the highest degree the natural ability to make their care acceptable to the patient. As in other forms of art, a natural talent can be encouraged and trained: but the tone-deaf will never be able to play the violin. It is the regrettable fact that there are doctors in hospital practice who will never be able to address their patients (or their students) except *de haut en bas*. They may well practice excellent medicine; but recognition of their skill is accorded only with reluctance and in qualified terms. Between the two extremes lie most of us who can achieve by practice a modest competence in communication which is sufficient for our needs. Whereas the patient does not choose his role, the practitioner in medicine does. He or she is therefore under a greater obligation to learn the skill of communication with the sick which lies at the heart of the matter.

When we are well it is hard to imagine what we feel like when sick. The healthy mind discards all but the outlines of an episode of sickness, recording the time and the fact of illness but dissolving the sensations of pain and misery. Ivan Illich in his destructive book *Medical Nemesis* seems to suggest that pain is ennobling and that doctors by reducing it or taking it away have somehow diminished the human experience. One wonders if he has ever suffered the pain which becomes an overmastering pre-occupation to the exclusion of all other mental processes, thus reducing the sufferer to the lowest ebb of human existence. The capacity required of the good doctor or nurse is to be able to imagine themselves in the patient's place.

There are both doctors and patients who engage in this most delicate of relationships without giving a thought to the problems and anxieties of each other. It is of course right for a doctor or nurse not to become emotionally involved with a patient's suffering, because that may distort their judgment. But that is not the same thing as egocentricity. Clinical detachment may take the form of a frigid pride in the technicalities of the art, in professional recognition, and in the widely-read publication. The patient may be equally self-centred, thinking of himself as the principal concern of the doctor; and of his aches, pains, and business disruption as unique in human experience. Between these extremes lies a wide range of failures in sympathy and communication which diminish the quality of care the patient receives. The allocation of blame for these failures was the principal task of the Health Service Commissioner and it fell sometimes on one party to the relationship and sometimes on the other, occasionally on both or neither.

*     *     *

To say that all patients should receive the best clinical care of which their attendants are capable is to state a banality. To say that patients must be made to believe they are getting it is more contentious. Not much observation of the human race is needed to learn that men and women act more in reliance on what they perceive to be facts than on the truth. If politics and advertising both depend on perception rather than truth, that is to denigrate neither but to recognize the practical limits to human understanding. In any case truth is of all concepts the most elusive. Salvador de Madariaga ends one of his novels with the words: 'Truth . . . truth . . . the aroma of a bunch of errors.'[2]

One of the doctor's many dilemmas is that the delivery of good clinical care may require a measure of deceit. That is the foundation of the placebo effect, the truth and validity of which is not in doubt. Indeed, pleasing the patient comes near to being as important as treating him skilfully and a vital ingredient in the effective delivery of health care as opposed to merely prescribing it. The patients of a doctor and the clients of an advocate all have a very clear mental image of how their advisers should look and speak. Failure to conform to the perceived stereotype induces immediate anxiety in patient or client. Nor is it of the slightest consequence that the person being advised or treated may hold strong political views about the unfair dominance of the professions or is of the criminal fraternity which mocks and affects to despise the law-abiding.

2. *A Bunch of Errors*, Jonathan Cape, 1954.

Whenever they are in trouble, they expect and may vociferously demand that their professional adviser looks the part and the confidence which that appearance inspires is an important element in the delivery of good care. This is not to say that an occasional stepping out of character will damage the proper relationship; on the contrary, the sudden appearance of familiar faces surmounting sweat-shirt and jeans, having hurried into hospital to cope with some dire emergency, may actually enhance the perception of basic humanity and goodness. But a return to normal formality on Monday morning will be expected.

*       *       *

A curiously fleeting but intimate example of the relationship is that between patient and anaesthetist. It is to this person that we surrender our consciousness and to whose power to make us totally vulnerable we voluntarily submit. His or hers is usually the last voice heard before embarking on what feels like a leap from a height into darkness. Some anaesthetists seem to think that theirs is a purely technological contribution to treatment, although none the less important for that. But the need to feel confidence and trust in the anaesthetist is sharply felt by the patient. The more knowledgeable the patient, the more sharply will the need be felt, because the patient will know how much he depends on the anaesthetist's care and skill to preserve his faculties during what may be several hours of oblivion on a reduced supply of oxygen.

A pre-operation visit which consists of more than a brief and formal consultation and routine questioning is immensely reassuring. That does not mean that the visit need be long. It is the manner of conducting it which will make the difference between clinical competence and good practice. I return to this topic later in connection with intensive care.

The quality of these relationships can be monitored only by those engaged in the delivery of care. It is of course true that some hospitals acquire a general reputation for the warmth with which they receive and greet their patients. But this general repute is impossible to measure and its loss may be so gradual as to be imperceptible. The truth is that our attitudes to one another, both privately and professionally, can be monitored only by self-examination. To do this honestly and effectively is very difficult. Nor are one's family or other immediate entourage reliable guides. Whether they love you or fear you, they will not be able to give a truthful answer to the question: 'What am I really like these days?'

It is sad but true that human beings tend to lack insight into their own characters and especially into defects of ability or temperament. I have known of instances in which a consultant of great experience and, it must be admitted, no inconsiderable age, earnestly believed that he possessed in the highest degree the ability to communicate with his patients effectively by 'talking to them straight from the shoulder—I find they like it.' He deduced this from the docile, or perhaps wooden, submissiveness of his patients in the face of observations which they regarded as nothing short of brutal. In subsequent confidences, these patients described the doctor's attitude as rude, abrasive and insensitive.[3] No doubt there are patients whose strength of character is such that complete candour is welcome to them. But there are as many others who are by nature timorous and need to absorb information gradually and with the help of familiar euphemisms. The art of communication lies in the accurate estimation of the temperament, strength and intelligence of the particular patient one is confronting at a given moment. No general rule or practice will suffice: each case requires to be considered on its own. To say that is of course to make great demands on very busy people and it may be a counsel of perfection which can seldom

3. For a much worse, indeed shocking, example of insensitivity and lack of insight, see C. M. FLETCHER: *Communication in Medicine,* Nuffield Provincial Hospitals Trust, 1973, p.13.

be followed. Yet if the delivery of health care is almost as important as its clinical content, the effectiveness of communication must be attended to.

An important component of the special relationship between doctor or nurse and patient is its confidentiality. The patient expects to be able to confide in considerable secrecy to his medical attendants the symptoms and feelings of his or her illness. It is an important part of communicating with the patient to gain this confidence and to retain it. I deal with this difficult and delicate topic at greater length in the First Digression below.

## THE FIRST DIGRESSION

Confidentiality in medicine has been the subject in recent times of declarations more passionate than reasonable. One perceives a strange tendency towards absolutism in a field where pragmatism is plainly more appropriate. For there are obviously many situations in which a doctor may find his moral and social duty overwhelmingly in favour of disclosure rather than concealment.

Must not the employer of an airline pilot or even a bus-driver be warned when a patient in one of those and perhaps many other occupations, complains of dizzy spells or some other more untoward symptom? Should not the spouse of a patient diagnosed as having a sexually transmissible disease be warned? I take it that every doctor would answer 'Yes' to those two questions. Yet there are other questions only a little less devastating in their implications to which I believe some doctors would answer differently. I have, for example, heard tell of an instance in which doctors refused to help police trying to identify a wounded robber who had mercilessly blasted an innocent person with a shotgun on the ground that because the robber had been treated in an Accident &

Emergency Department, the confidential relationship of doctor and patient had arisen and imposed a duty of silence.[4] I have direct knowledge of the refusal of disclosure of medical records which could prove or disprove the truth of allegations of criminal conduct made against police officers. To declare that an absolute duty of confidence arises merely from the relationship existing between the casualty officer of the day and a man seeking treatment for a gunshot wound on a single occasion, seems to me to fly in the face of common sense as well as to disregard a social duty.

Moreover, the extent to which doctors are willing to give non-medical persons, or medically qualified people having no relationship with the patient, ready access to case-notes makes a logical nonsense of the absolutist position. Such disclosure sometimes extends to social workers whose connection with the medical aspects of a case is tenuous. In fact the potential for leakage of confidential information in the hospital service is massive. Such leakage was a not uncommon cause of complaint to me in the office of Health Service Commissioner.

The law's view of the matter is, I suggest, admirably practical. The technical language of the law groups these problems of disclosure of confidence under the heading of 'Privilege', that is to say, a law or right which is private and special to a person or situation. One of these privileges is the right to keep hidden, or sometimes to disclose without penalty, facts which might help the discovery of truth. The fundamental rule is that justice is so important to everyone in the orderly resolution of the conflicts which arise in society, that its interests are paramount and that no information should therefore be kept from a court of law.

The only absolute and unqualified privilege against disclo-

---

4. For a recent example of medical confusion of thought, see the incident reported in the *Daily Telegraph* of 15 September 1987, where it was said that a London hospital refused to help the police identify a mugger who used a broken bottle as a weapon and later sought treatment for a cut thumb.

sure of confidential oral and written exchanges is legal professional privilege, that is to say, the right of lawyers to keep from a court all oral or written matter which has passed between them and their clients in connection with the litigation. Even as I write, I can sense the hackles of my medically qualified readers rising. But once the initial thought that the lawyers have been favouring themselves is succeeded by a deeper consideration, it is obvious that the judicial process as we know it in this country would be impossible without such a privilege. For it would then be open to counsel for either side to a dispute to call as a witness the legal advisers on the other—including his opponent colleague. The questions to be asked would include what the client actually said when he first took advice, what advice was given, what risks in the litigation were foreseen, which witnesses were thought unreliable or dangerous to call and many others of a like kind. The duty to answer such questions truthfully and to tell the *whole* truth would make it virtually impossible for clients to take legal advice. I would not like to be obliged to repeat in court all that doctor-clients have told me in bygone litigation.

It follows that there is no such thing as an absolute medical professional privilege against disclosure of a patient's affairs, any more than there is such a thing as the 'Seal of the Confessional'. Both the doctor and the priest will be held in contempt of court if they refuse to answer a relevant and important question in litigation on the ground that to do so would breach medical or spiritual confidence. That this state of the law has produced not a single instance of a doctor or priest being sent to prison for refusing to answer questions, a 'contempt of court', is attributable to the good sense and goodwill of all the professions concerned. The good doctor knows well enough when his moral and social duty requires that he should breach a confidence for a greater good: and judges never press a doctor or a priest for answers to confidential questions which the issues in the litigation before them do not absolutely require.

So a practical solution has served us well. Although I know of no instance in which a doctor or priest has been committed to prison for refusing to answer a question in court, a journalist has.[5] Many doctors, hospital administrators and others protect themselves from accusations of breach of confidence by requiring that an order of the court for production be obtained before they disclose confidential matters. Although this may sometimes unreasonably increase the cost and time taken up in obtaining evidence, one can understand the motive. It is embarrassing to be wrongly accused of breaching confidence, but there should be no embarrassment in obeying the order of a court.[6]

One strange and, to a lawyer, interesting complication in this field arises from the very existence of a National Health Service. Someone has to be the owner of its vast properties, consisting of both estates and chattels. That someone is deemed to be the Secretary of State who notionally owns every hypodermic needle and every dressing.

It follows that he owns the various forms of card and paper (and nowadays probably magnetic tape and film as well) upon which are recorded by handwriting or other means, information about patients much of which is confidential in nature. Since he owns the substance of the material on which the record is inscribed, he is inclined to say, on the advice of lawyers, that he owns the information as well.

This raises a beautiful problem for lawyers, the more beautiful because of its nakedness, unclothed as it is in much practical importance. The Romans got to it first. What, they asked themselves, happens when an artist paints a picture on someone else's board or, more pertinently, someone writes a poem on another person's paper? No doubt in those days both

---

5. A–G v Mulholland (1963) 2 QB 477.

6. This procedure has received some statutory sanction under Section 12 of the Police and Criminal Evidence Act 1984 which obliges the police to obtain an order from a judge for access to medical records for the purposes of a criminal investigation; but having obtained the order, they may seize the documents.

board and paper were relatively scarcer and more valuable than they are today. Who owns the resultant object? The answers to the question were in general favourable to the base materialism of mankind:

Litterae quoque, licet aureae sint, perinde chartis membranisque cedunt . . . ideoque si in chartis membranisve tuis carmen vel historiam vel orationem Titius scripserit, huius corporis non Titius sed tu dominus esse iudiceris.[7]

This runs counter to the argument that by exercising professional skill and art on a blank form, the doctor turns it into something different, a creation of which he is the rightful owner. It is possible that in Justinian's day[8] the materials on which one wrote were more valuable by scarcity than anything one could inscribe upon them. Yet in another passage, Justinian writes:

If someone were to paint a picture on another person's board, there are those to whom it seems that the picture becomes part of the board. But to us it seems better that the board should become part of the picture; for it is absurd that a painting by Apelles or Parrhasius should become part of a cheap board.[9]

The Romans argued amongst themselves about the justice of these two ideas and the apparent inconsistency between them. But they made provision anyway for the payment by the writer or artist to the owner of the paper or board of their value, which could not be refused, after which ownership passed to the craftsman, unless there had been bad faith.

There is plainly an available argument for doctors that by exercising the skills of their art upon paper provided by the Secretary of State for their use, they become the owners of the

7. *Justinian's Institutes* Book II, Title I, 33. A rough translation would be: 'Lettering also, even of gold, in the same way becomes part of papers or parchments . . . and therefore if Titius were to write a poem, or a story or a speech on your papers or parchments, you and not Titius would be judged to be the owner of this object.'
8. A.D. 533
9. Ibid. 34. Apelles and Parrhasius were great portrait painters of their day.

resultant documents just as they are the owners of any notes they bring into existence about patients whom they treat privately. On the other hand, where a doctor is employed expressly for the purpose of creating patient records for use by his employer, for example in a factory carrying on some dangerous process or in a pharmaceutical company, it seems right that the ownership of the records should remain with the employer. And there can be instances of the patient seeming to own the results of special investigations, e.g. X-rays, separately and privately paid for.

\*      \*      \*

One further aspect of medical notes deserves passing attention because it was the subject of frequent complaint to the Health Service Commissioner that a patient had been badly or unfairly dealt with. This is the vexed question of access for patients to their own medical notes.

In the many words which have been written on this topic, mostly in an emotional vein, it is seldom that the proper distinction is made between records of fact and records of opinion. Quite apart from personal details, which may embrace such matters as religious belief or lack of it and previous hospital admissions, most hospital notes contain a mass of factual material ranging from X-rays to blood analyses, much of which will be meaningless to the patient without skilled help to interpret it. There seems little reason to deny the average patient access to this material for what it is worth to him. He may even be able to correct a damaging mistake of fact, for example that he had been imprisoned for a time or had been admitted to a mental hospital, both of which misfortunes have on occasion been wrongly attributed to patients due to similarities of name or the like error. There may be occasions when even a statement of fact, for example the record of surgery to remove a tumour, may be undesirable knowledge for a sensitive patient and those treating him

A Special Relationship

should be entitled to the last word on that. But such things apart, it is difficult to see that much harm could flow from giving patients access to purely factual information in their notes. Some good might even result from patients appreciating at last what so few of them understand, namely, the enormous amount of skill and care which goes into dealing with their problems.

It is a very different matter to give patients access to statements of opinion. There is not just the problem of the hopeless prognosis. Doctors and nurses are bound to record not only their assessments of the temperament, mood, and courage of their patients but also of their truthfulness and propensity for good or evil, their relationship with family and friends, and a wide range of other judgments which are matters purely of personal opinion. Such judgments may be very wounding even when accurate and more so if deemed by the patient to be inaccurate. I do not think it would be practicable to confer on patients a right of access to such material, without seriously endangering the relationship between doctor and patient or nurse and patient. Neither would feel free to write their candid and spontaneous beliefs about diagnosis, current status, and prognosis of patients if they knew that there was a legal right to study those opinions either during the time of admission or subsequently. Such an intolerable inhibition of personal expression could lead only to a lower standard of treatment. Important observations or speculations about a patient's condition would either go unrecorded or be driven underground to some private and unofficial notebook of unusual cases, more likely the former.

The virtually insoluble problem is that fact and opinion are not easily separable in case notes. Some records, such as X-ray films themselves, ECGs, blood analyses, and the like are separate items which could be segregated in a distinct pocket of the medical notes. But very commonly they are accompanied, and need to be, by an expression of expert opinion on their proper interpretation. To separate one from the other would be to make the notes less useful and less accessible to those who most have to use them.

All professions need to be able to record in some private and confidential place, their innermost thoughts about the affairs of their clients. This is certainly true of lawyers, accountants, and bankers and must be equally true of doctors. All these advisers need to be confident that their good relationship with their clients will not be damaged by disclosure of an occasional critical or adverse judgment which is not intended to wound or to damage the client's affairs, but to help in the proper conduct of them. Experience in those countries which have enthusiastically embraced total freedom of information (Sweden, for example) tends to show that the really vital information about people and their affairs gradually disappears from records of opinion, which become more and more sterile and perfunctory and for that reason less useful. I hope that the authorities in this country will think long and carefully before embarking upon any scheme for opening case notes to the inspection of patients or, worse still, those purporting to act on their behalf. There are no doubt some patients whose fundamentally healthy constitution and disposition may make it harmless and even instructive or amusing for them to browse through their own notes. Let their medical advisers be the judges of that.

Reverting finally to the observation that complaints to the Health Service Commissioner about patients' notes were quite common, it is interesting to consider the motivation of many of these complaints. The desire to see the notes was often matched by a strong determination to have them amended to conform more closely with the patient's opinion of what they should have said. There was sometimes discernible, I thought, an Orwellian desire to alter the course of history retrospectively. Unpleasant events or opinions should be made as if they had never happened or been held. The use of words like 'expunge' or 'expurgate' often seemed to underline the complainant's urge to re-write the past. One particular complainant dwells in my memory. He wished the entry '? aggressive psychopath' to be 'expunged' from his notes (which had been carelessly left within his reach) and threatened to visit all manner of violent retribution on everyone concerned if this were not done.

These observations in no way derogate from the doctor's and the nurse's bounden duty to write truthful and fair, as opposed to loose and malicious, comments in their patients' notes. This duty was not, in my experience, always observed as it should have been. The consequences of unfair comment in a patient's notes may be far-reaching and may severely damage his or her acceptability to the profession. If notes are to remain the inviolable repository of medical confidence, then the duty of fairness must be raised proportionately, to the highest standard and must be rigorously observed.

# 2
# Contented Travaillers

'When I was at home, I was in a better place,
but travellers must be content.'
Shakespeare, *A.Y.L.* II iv 18.

The single episode of acute illness is the commonest occasion
calling for medical intervention. The majority of people
attaining middle-age will have experienced one such episode
of greater or less importance. Assuming an admission while
conscious, such an episode resembles a journey at the start of
which one is seen off by family or friends but which is
essentially a journey amongst strangers. To the stress and
uncertainty of illness are therefore added the pressures of
meeting and establishing relations with persons previously
unknown. Sundry incidental discomforts are experienced as
the journey goes on.

The arrival at the point of departure is of great importance
to the morale of the patient. How the heart sinks on first
seeing a new place of work, some temporary accommodation,
or the hospital in which one is to undergo a wholly new
experience! 'First depressions on arrival', wrote Sir Osbert
Sitwell with a perfect perception of this human frailty. It is at
the point of departure on the journey that the delivery of care
depends on the administrator. There can be no underestimat-
ing the importance to the perception of care which good
administration can make. In a good hospital someone comes
forward to receive the arriving patient, takes his bag and utters
some words to the effect that the patient is both expected and
welcome. He then leads off the patient and any companion
without hesitation in the right direction. By contrast, patients
quite often have the experience of not being expected owing
to some oversight, not being at all welcome for the same

reason, and having to wait while some temporary accommodation is found. The morale sinks at each of these impediments.

Reception on the ward is a continuation of the process, but the stresses on the patient increase. There may be the scrutiny, open or surreptitious, of other patients to be suffered, perhaps followed by the unnatural process of getting undressed in the middle of the day and climbing into bed. It is not possible to remove these nervous apprehensions because the circumstances giving rise to them are real. But it is possible to minimize their effect by the kindness with which the necessary instructions are given. Some nurses have little idea of how chill, forbidding, and detached their professional voices sound. Once again the apparent coolness is more probably due to a lack of imagination than to any lack of natural warmth.

\*  \*  \*

There was a time, not so long ago, when it was usual to spread straw on the road outside the house in which someone was ill. This tended to deaden the sound of horses' hooves and the iron tyres of cartwheels. So it must have been very generally supposed that people when sick find noise unpleasant. Perhaps it interferes with the brief spells of daytime sleep which is all the very sick can sometimes achieve. But it may equally be a low-grade discomfort to the wakeful.

This simple observation seems in many hospitals today to have been forgotten. Complaints of noise on the ward were a recurrent feature of complaints to the Health Service Commissioner. The Nightingale ward is obviously the place where the nuisance of noise is most oppressive. A very common cause of the trouble is the failure of the administration to maintain the hospital radio receiving equipment in proper working order or to see that the bedside units function correctly. This failure leads the patients to resort to using their personal radios, often to the great discomfort of their neighbours. Nursing staff, who are commonly young and fit, may find this acceptable or even congenial. It is nowadays possible to listen to personal radio or tape-reproduction equipment through headphones of excellent quality. The endlessly twittering television set in the corner, to which no one is really paying attention, is another potent source of discomfort.

A restless and unhappy patient responds less well to treatment, however good it may be. It is therefore an important element in the delivery of good health care to maintain a calm and restful environment on the ward in which each patient can peacefully suffer the burden of illness in the way which seems best to him or her. Noise is as perceptible a form of pollution as a dirty floor, so that for once it is a simple matter for those whose business it is to monitor this important failing.

*     *     *

A great deal of nonsense is talked about lack of sleep in hospitals. I fear that much of it may be expressed by those who have either never been seriously ill or have been admitted to hospital for studies or observation only. It is seldom that people ill enough to be admitted to and retained in hospital can take much exercise. They very commonly take a rest or short sleep in the early afternoon and are encouraged to do so. Night comes on rather earlier than is usual, often at or about 10 o'clock. Most of those who are really ill sleep only fitfully. For them, the sound of the six o'clock teacups in preparation may be a delightful relief. Some even find that they sleep or doze more successfully in the ensuing two hours after the refreshment of tea and sympathy which morning has brought. If patients are able after an average day in hospital to sleep from 10.30 p.m. until 8 o'clock the following morning, the probability is that it is time they were sent home. The solution to this problem is essentially a professional one which it would be impertinent in me to try to solve. There may, for example be considerations on an orthopaedic ward which differ markedly from those on a medical or general surgical ward and that account must be taken of these differences. All I can say is that a very sick person does not want the night extended and that I do not recall a single complaint to the Health Service Commissioner of being woken too early.

\*     \*     \*

Mealtimes are generally looked forward to by patients with an enthusiasm which their feeble appetite disappoints. It is not the fault of the food, which is necessarily of the kind sometimes described as 'institutional'. This means that it is prepared in the most difficult circumstances for the most difficult of customers. There are many by whom the notion that food ought to be very hot in order to be good for you is stoutly held. It is enormously difficult to achieve this requirement in most hospitals, but perhaps it is a comfort which administrators should try to provide if only to encourage patients to eat at a time when they may need to do so but are little inclined.

One curious omission is to be noticed in the catering arrangements of a great many hospitals and that is the failure to provide sufficient dietary fibre at a time when the recumbent and inactive patient most needs it. It is difficult or impossible for the patient who ordinarily takes fibre daily in cereal form on first eating in the morning to obtain what he requires, usually in greater amounts than he would customarily need. Again there are those for whom the patient's diet is a professional responsibility and I must ask to be forgiven for even mentioning the matter. But it may be that what is prescribed and what actually reaches the wards are two different things and that here too there is a need for continuous monitoring of what is happening at the point of delivery.

\*      \*      \*

NOT FAMOUS, NOT LAST . . .

The law relating to offences against the person has always distinguished between those assaults in which the skin is broken and those in which it is not. Thus a blow to the body which does grievous bodily harm without breaking the continuity of the skin is treated with some severity: but it is treated as altogether different in character from the class of offences described as 'wounding' in which the skin is broken. This is in general regarded as the more serious category, no doubt because the integrity of the skin is instinctively recognized as important or perhaps because the spilling of blood is involved in the one category and not visibly in the other. The patient's fundamental apprehension of his treatment is conditioned, perhaps unconsciously, by the same considerations. Oral medication he undergoes by his own act of more or less free will. But a breaking of the skin must generally be done to him. It is of course a question of degree. The intramuscular and even the intravenous injection is so small an interference with physical integrity that it causes no real apprehension in the average patient, although there are a few for whom even that minimal assault produces an uncontrollable reflex, often to their own great embarrassment.

An operation of intermediate or major degree, however, is another matter. It is doubtful if any patient contemplates that degree of interference without some measure of anxiety. Preparation for such an event is therefore an important part of the delivery of health care.

Warning the patient of what to expect after recovery is standard practice in good hospitals and where the planned intervention will involve a stay in the ITU, of obvious importance. Patients who have just undergone the planned procedure and are recovering well, may be useful in re-assuring those who are waiting their turn. They are usually very willing to undertake this small work of mercy. It is perhaps trite to observe that what is essential is to build up the patient's confidence in the ability of the operation to make him better than he is at the moment.

What may be less commonly recognized is that once a patient has been told that an operation is the recommended treatment, he begins instinctively to brace himself to face what he imagines, with varying accuracy, to be an ordeal. When confronted with a danger which has to be faced, the man or woman of ordinary resolution will want to advance to meet it. Some may flee, by refusing the offered procedure. But few will want to stand still.

From this cause flows one of the commonest complaints about the delivery of health care—the postponed operation. To a degree which only he fully understands, the patient prepares himself to meet with dignity and cheerfulness an event of which he may be, despite his denials, mortally afraid. At the least he will be conscious of an occasion which calls for courage and composure. As the patient reaches the crest of this wave of preparatory effort, it is quite commonly and casually announced to him that his name has been taken out of the list. To those who see hundreds of operating lists and the patients on them come and go in the course of a year, this event is of little significance. To the patient, it comes as a severe blow to the morale. It is not merely that the danger that he was willing to confront has stepped back so that he cannot now come to grips with it. The damage is more far-reaching than that. The patient knows that his ultimate recovery is further away and that he must make the effort to summon up his courage all over again. Curiously, one of the worst aspects of postponement is the sense of having failed in some way: the visiting family and friends must be told that after all the heroic day of encounter is not to take place, although it may be reinstated on some unspecified day in the future: and their anxieties are prolonged. The patient may have evolved, after long thought, a few suitable phrases in which to express his love and concern for his dependents and his determination to recover. These famous last words are not delivered: they are neither famous, nor last.

\*      \*      \*

On a first occasion, this experience for the patient is no more than a disappointment, although it may be a severe one. But subsequent second, third, or even further postponements may reduce even the most resolute patient to despair.

There are obvious reasons of emergency which make this kind of hardship unavoidable. The first thing to do, therefore, is to explain the nature of that emergency to the patient, so that he may feel that his own unhappiness is suffered in a good cause. The next comfort to be given is the reassurance that his operation remains a matter of priority and that his name will be back in the list at the earliest opportunity.

It sometimes seems as if operating lists deliberately include patients who are very likely either to be taken out of the list late on the same day or not to be reached on the operating day for want of time and staff. It is understandable that lists should be well-filled, given the long waiting time which prevails in many specialties. But it should always be remembered that every patient taken out of an operating list is one made to suffer a considerable further burden in the course of his illness.

The period of waiting for treatment is anyway a testing one for patients and they often suffer from feelings of despair that they make no progress towards recovery and that they are a useless burden to their families and to those in hospital who care for them. These feelings can be relieved by skilled and sensitive communication. To one such patient who expressed dismay at idle, unprogressive, and useless days, a young nurse said 'You are just at the beginning of a long journey. You should take all the rest you can get.' This has always seemed to me the perfect example of nursing communication. The analogy used was such as would at one stroke make the patient feel less useless and more to be respected: and make him see the waiting days as an active preparation for a necessary and worthy endeavour lying ahead.

\*       \*       \*

Intensive care is increasingly used as surgical and anaesthetic technology advances and the need for close support in the recovery period becomes more common. The technology is immensely impressive not least to the patient, if and when he becomes aware of it.

To some patients the awareness of total dependency in intensive care is disturbing and unpleasant. Much depends on the temperament of the individual. The more proud and self-centred they are, the more likely are they to resent instinctively the total surrender involved. It may be that with these patients the liberal use of sedatives is the only solution, although they will suffer the longer for it afterwards.

But there are others for whom the realization of dependence brings with it a joy of recognition and gratitude which make the experience of intensive care happily memorable. To be thus completely in the hands of other human beings is an experience which few will have had since childhood, of which they have little recollection. The warmth, the nakedness, the inability to speak, and the limitations of movement are all characteristics of infancy. To experience them again, but this time with a mature mind and without the maternal bond, can be unpleasant unless a good mutual relationship is established between nurse and patient.

Given the right communication between two right-minded people, a period of intensive care can be recalled with deep feelings of satisfaction. In the first place, I sometimes wonder if nurses are sufficiently alert to the extent to which sedated patients can hear and understand what is being said and, indeed, remember it afterwards. It is important not only to refrain from saying things which may seem unfeeling or disrespectful of the patient, but actively to talk to them even when they cannot reply.

Touch is also important. When we meet people for the first time, or meet them again after any considerable absence, we are accustomed to clasp one another's hands. Some nations make this physical contact on a first meeting each day. The handclasp is an instant of warmth and reassurance.

Patients in intensive care may like their hand to be taken occasionally and warmly pressed or to have a hand laid on the shoulder, simply for the pleasure of human contact which that brings.

It is of course a matter not for me but for professional judgment: but I sometimes wonder if patients are not too heavily sedated as a matter of routine in some intensive care units. I have wondered if spells of greater consciousness during daytime would not be welcomed by many such patients having the right temperament. The reduction of their overall intake of sedative drugs would be reduced and that could only be beneficial. But they would derive also the great psychological benefit that comes with recognition of the faces of those who are caring for them and of some degree of communication with them, even if not by speech.

Of course those whose pain or distress is such that they become restless and anxious on perceiving their condition must simply be sedated until those reactions disappear. They are unlucky. I merely suggest that patients in intensive care should be cautiously allowed occasional periods of greater awareness in which to perceive an experience which may be worth remembering for those who can see the positive side of it.

\*     \*     \*

There is an inclination in some hospitals to make the patients in an open ward share their mealtimes at a common table. This is no doubt a good idea for those who by temperament and degree of recovery are suited to it. But it should never, I suggest, be made a matter of compulsion. There is already in the fact of admission to hospital, a serious loss of privacy and independence. To be made to eat communally, as if at school or in prison, is a further and needless deprivation of personal freedom. Patients will soon enough join together to share meals if their inclination and compatibility of temperament prompt them to it; and the sharing will be the happier for the extended invitation and its acceptance. Others will, while still sick, prefer to tackle their meals alone and will join in communal activities when ready.

Joint remedial classes may often produce the same unhappy effect and should be avoided unless staffing needs make it impossible, when the class should be made voluntary. Nothing is more humiliating to mature adults who happen to be suffering from some common disability, than to oblige them to swing their arms or attempt to walk in unison. There will often be an unhappy contrast between the physical states and capabilities of individuals within the group.

\*  \*  \*

Another disagreeable aspect of life on the ward is the oppressive visitor. Some patients, by ill-luck or bad arrangement, sustain a surfeit of noisy and demonstrative visitors at every visiting hour, commandeering every chair and dominating the ward with conversation and jocularity to the great discomfort of others. It should not be permitted to happen and need not be. A firm but tactful word of reminder that some patients are really quite ill and need rest and quiet should suffice.

Not every doctor or nurse realizes what an effort the patient puts forth to welcome and reassure his visitors. It is a natural reaction of the mentally healthy patient. Consider the behaviour of one who stumbles or slips on ice and falls. Good citizens will come to help him to his feet, the first and most essential need, as has already been remarked. In response to expressions of concern he will often assert quite wrongly that he is 'perfectly all right' or will be so 'in a minute or two'. The disinclination to admit defeat is very powerful.

So it is that when visitors come, the patient instinctively does his best to reassure them that he is either not really ill at all or is much recovered. And he will make the usual and appropriate enquiries about the continuing and normal lives of his visitors, their friends and relations. The effort of doing this may leave the patient damp with perspiration and, if the visit is prolonged, quite exhausted. Visitors should be waylaid and warned of this problem. Perhaps they should also be reminded that the question 'Am I tiring you?' is pointless and insensitive, because it is almost impossible to answer it truthfully. If the patient wants a particular visitor to stay longer, he will make that known soon enough. If visitors are not asked to stay when they politely say that they must go, it is because the patient knows that he has had enough and must, perhaps regretfully, let his visitors go and return once more to the essentially lonely business of getting better.

\*     \*     \*

I suppose doctors and surgeons try to visit their patients as often as their busy days will permit. But I doubt if they can imagine what reassurance their visits give to the patients, or how anxiously they are awaited or how disappointed patients are when the anticipated visit does not occur. Even a very short visit is better than none, especially if the right words of sympathy and encouragement are found. The worst neglect of all is to pass by the bed of the patient who is expected shortly to die and for whom not much can be done. This does still happen from time to time.

Those who have never been in such a position will also find it hard to imagine how curious and unhappy are the patient's sensations when the visit takes the form of a teaching round.

Then the patient must try to look agreeable and interested in face of a group of people who manifestly see him only as a case of more or less professional interest. The detached conversation about him, in which he is hardly ever invited to join, is disconcerting to the point of embarrassment. Although most patients of goodwill would consent to the presence of students if asked, in fact they seldom are. They make the best of a bad episode by offering jocular replies intended to put everyone at ease, an effort in which they are all too often unsuccessful, as their group of visitors clearly indicate by their faces.

This is a phase in human relations which it is extremely difficult for either party to carry off well. Admittedly, these visits must take place if the next generation of doctors and nurses is to learn. But I believe they could nearly always be better managed than they are. I acknowledge at once that some doctors and surgeons, whose particular skill in communication I have already commended, deal with the situation extremely well, involving the patient as well as the students in the discussion and making him feel rather that the whole group is concerned for his welfare, than that they are there only to learn by watching him. Such excellent doctors are, I suspect from complaints examined, more rare than they ought to be. Many could do better at this task by simply trying harder.

In the first place, I think it may be easier for patients if doctor and students come close alongside them. It is certainly more disconcerting to be gazed at from the foot of the bed, as an interesting animal may be studied in captivity.

If possible, the technical language should be kept for a later discussion over the case-notes. It is again unhappy for the patient to have to listen to an animated discussion which he knows to be about himself but of which he can understand only the odd word. To use technical jargon in his presence is as ill-mannered towards him as it is to speak a foreign language at the dinner table knowing that the principal guest does not understand it.

Much depends, too, on a proper estimation of the patient's own intelligence and ability to understand his illness. This calculation could with advantage be made at the time of the first examination on admission and even recorded on the notes by some system of grading. The patient could then be drawn more or less into the teaching discussion as seems appropriate. Many highly intelligent patients have been insulted by off-hand treatment in these circumstances. If they have been well educated, they will instantly recognize the words of Latin or Greek derivation and, alas, the awful hybrids. They will understand perfectly the difference between hypertension and hypotension, apnoea and dyspnoea. Most regrettably of all, their esteem for doctors who have been unable to detect that their patient understands most of what is being said, or who care about it not at all, will fall drastically: they may even come to regard them with tolerant amusement or, ultimately, with contempt. This cannot be good for the relationship of doctor and patient and therefore ultimately for the patient's recovery.

All that I have offered for consideration in the preceding paragraphs applies with equal force to nurses, subject to the appropriate substitutions. The commonest offenders in this respect are the two nurses required for some purpose to work together from either side of the same bed. The situation has so often been depicted both comically and critically on film or television, that I need not labour the offence which insensitive conversation may give.

\* \* \*

Failure to communicate properly within the hospital is of course a potent source of dissatisfaction with the service, no matter how good the medical care may be. Incorrect medication or dosage are fairly obvious, though regrettably frequent, results of lapses in clear communication. One common form of this failure is that patient A receives the medicine destined for patient B and vice versa. It is a somewhat wry observation that I never once heard that such a mistake had harmed a patient. Presumably the mistake was seldom persisted in and everyone can tolerate a small dose of practically anything. Wrong dosage, on the other hand is usually disastrous; one of the commonest and most lethal is an adult dose for an infant, closely followed in dangerous potential by a wrong dose of insulin.

Another manifestation of failure in communication is the attempt to examine patient A with the aid of the medical records of patient B. The attempt is not usually persisted in for long and it is rare for this to harm anyone. But it is apt to fray the tempers of all parties affected by the mistake. Other failures produce episodes of black comedy. In Vienna a young man in perfect health went to visit a friend in hospital. On entering, he slipped on a wet floor, fell and fractured his femur. He was undressed and put on a trolley to go for X-ray. And there, disastrously, he was left unattended and unlabelled. Presently the doors of a nearby operating theatre swung open, porters emerged and wheeled the young man into the theatre, whence he emerged some time later having had a pace-maker fitted. He suffered no lasting harm.

Other episodes are more macabre and less amusing. Infective hepatitis is of course an extremely dangerous disease to have in a hospital and energetic measures to isolate victims and to prevent the spread of the infection are fully justified. But one must first accurately establish that the disease is present if one is to take certain drastic steps. A man arrived dead at a particular hospital, having suffered a collapse from some heart condition. He had three years previously been treated in another hospital for infective hepatitis of which he had been completely cured, as his records showed. By some failure in communication on the telephone between the two hospitals, the second hospital decided that the dead man still presented a risk of infection, which was quite positively not the case.

Thereupon, a sequence of bizarre happenings ensued. The unhappy widow's house was fumigated from top to bottom, a process which killed all her house-plants. The dead man's clothing and possessions, including a useful sum of money, were incinerated. Finally, the deceased's coffin was presented to the widow for the funeral with four-inch wide strips of vivid yellow adhesive tape prominently affixed thereto bearing the legends in large capitals: 'DANGER OF INFECTION' and 'BURN WITHOUT OPENING'. Many readers will recognize these as merely some of the precautions which it is proper to take once the presence of this particular infection has been correctly identified. There is nothing outlandish about the precautions themselves. But in the first place there was no need for any of them and in the second place a sort of unreasoning panic seemed to set in which needlessly added to the widow's distress.[10]

It is an interesting observation of mishaps in hospital that they are very seldom the handiwork of one person alone. Most disasters are the result of a cascade of errors culminating in a mishap which there were several opportunities of preventing. It seems likely that this explains why failures in communication do not more often produce disaster—there is nearly always a chance of breaking into the sequence at some point and someone does so. It is only in rare instances that the initial error gets through the cascade to the end of the sequence, to produce a disastrous result.

The measurement of these and other aspects of the quality of care is extraordinarily difficult.[11] The quality sought is more likely to be the result of morale than of direction. Morale is sensed rather than measured, as every soldier knows. The collapse of morale exhales an aura as apparent to the

10. Case W585/84–85 H.S.C. Selected Investigations Oct 85–Mar 86 Cmnd. 440
11. In recent times attempts to do this scientifically have been made both here and in the United States, using the system called Qualpac. I understand that it is not yet in widespread use. But a reliable method of measuring the quality of care would of course be enormously useful.

sensitive manager as is the unusually scented breath of certain patients to the physician. The compelling necessity for the medical administrator or nurse-manager, as for the commanding officer, is to get away from the desk and go to where the fight is in progress. It requires self-discipline of a high order to do this as often as one should. The in-tray piled with apparently urgent matters is a discouragement to action. But the urgency of the paperwork is illusory in comparison with the need to maintain or restore morale at the front where the basic work of care goes on. It is again a curious feature of human relations that the appearance of the managers at the front matters far more than anything which they may subsequently do. There may not be much they can do; but their willingness to view the problem of the moment and to consider possible action to solve it raises hope and therefore morale.

# 3
# Convalescence

'How sickness enlarges the dimensions
of a man's self to himself!'
CHARLES LAMB, *The Convalescent.*

Patients who have undergone a successful operation, or been resuscitated by intensive care and then returned to the ward, or otherwise treated are in general going to get better. They may for that reason be less interesting professionally to both doctors and nurses. They are often allowed to feel that quite strongly.

This awareness of a depreciated status is a very common cause of complaint. The complaints which are made are often intrinsically of no merit. But the source from which they spring is the sense of depreciation and disregard.

The paradox here is that although the patient at this point of recovery has often been rescued from a premature death, he is actually feeling more ill and more in need of sympathy than at any previous time during his stay in hospital. All the benefits conferred on the patient by way of expert diagnosis and treatment may go unappreciated if the follow-up is neglected.

The accumulated effects of therapeutic, anaesthetic, analgesic, and sedative drugs are in some patients quite toxic. The patient will often feel extremely unwell in unspecific ways. It may be perfectly true that with the passing of time all these symptoms of pain and malaise will disappear harmlessly and without need for specific treatment. But if in addition the patient feels that he is now less deserving as an object of attention and sympathy, his morale will fall and he may later perceive this period of recovery as an episode of neglect.

There is a tendency also to disregard, or insufficiently attend to, the patient's complaints of minor illness unrelated to the major specialty which caused his admission. For example, patients who have had a serious operation followed by intensive care, commonly experience an inability to masticate food properly for some considerable time afterwards. Others suffer from severe constipation, fits of violent coughing, and minor injuries due to pressure or handling during unconsciousness. The discomfort these symptoms cause to the already debilitated patient may be quite disproportionate to their gravity. Neglected, they become potent sources of complaint even though they are not themselves in any way grave matters. Not to realize this and to take these matters seriously is a distinct failure in the delivery of health care which is liable to vitiate the good work previously done.

One sees very well how easy it is in a hard-pressed service to turn one's attention away from those who, although they feel temporarily far from well, are obviously going to recover quite soon. But what is required is less the delivery of any technical care than of an attitude which makes the patient feel that although on the mend he is still welcome in the hospital and not just a tiresome and professionally uninteresting burden. Once again, we encounter the crucial problem of communication, where what has to be conveyed is not factual matter but a sense of personal concern and interest.

*     *     *

When complaints about medical care are investigated far from the scene and time of occurrence, one of the remarkable features which emerge is the unawareness of staff that the patient was other than entirely contented. The better the patient, the more truly a *patient,* the less will he wish to articulate his feelings. There are many reasons for this.

In the first place, the vast majority of patients are profoundly grateful for the rescue operation which has been mounted on their behalf. To complain about any part of it seems ungrateful. So mordant is this feeling that even when patients do complain, they very commonly try to disclaim their grievance by asserting that they complain 'only so that others may not suffer as I did'. For my part, I did not always find this show of altruism convincing. In many cases which I studied as Health Service Commissioner, I simply did not believe it. But in fact there often was a legitimate cause for complaining and one which did deserve attention for the benefit of other patients. And a benefit for others is a very common outcome of a complaint which might not have been very well motivated initially.

In the second place, it is difficult to complain to the actual giver of care about his standard of care. To complain to the maker or seller of goods about the quality of his goods is difficult enough, involving as it does a confrontation which has an element of conflict in it. Such a confrontation is for most patients an impossible one to face. The patient is not only enfeebled at the time, but he feels at the disadvantage which I noted at the outset of this monograph.

When I came to investigate certain complaints about care, it was often said with indignation that the patient had uttered not a word of complaint about any aspect of his treatment at the time, as if that cast a doubt on all his later assertions. The very expression of such a protest betrays an alarming unawareness of the patient's predicament.

One of the more trying things for a patient is the need to ask nurses, who will often, perhaps usually, be much younger than he, for help in fundamental needs. He will usually try desperately to attend to these matters for himself. And when he cannot, he will notice the busy life of the nurses and defer asking for whatever he needs as long as possible. This will not be true of all patients some of whom will be tiresome, demanding, and self-centred persons. But I believe it will be true of the average decent person and of course the nursing staff will be the best judges of which of the patients fall into what category. The result is often that by the time the patient has brought himself to ask for attention, his need for whatever it is is fairly urgent. To leave him then unattended, his request often forgotten, is a common and distressful source of dissatisfaction, the more resented because the patient has tried, mistakenly perhaps, to avoid giving trouble and making work for people.

It is in fact at this stage in an episode of illness that the genesis of a complaint in the formal sense is most likely to take place. The patient is beginning to recover some of his physical normality and with it, regrettably, some of his aggressive instincts. He finds more to complain about and the energy to complain about it. And, as I have pointed out, he is apt to find himself less a centre of interest and to see that position usurped by more recent arrivals. Now is the time to quash the incipient complaint with a few diplomatic words of sympathy and interest, before it takes root, as unattended it certainly will. The chances are that at this stage of his recovery, the patient will be far more communicative, especially with his visiting relatives. By now he will be giving them graphic accounts of his remarkable sufferings and nigh miraculous recovery. At this point the patient or his relatives may well begin to find fault.

By no means do I suggest that the unreasonable and captious criticisms of the ill-natured and ungrateful patient or relative should be treated as if they were reasonable grounds for complaint. But where the patient or his family seem genuine enough, even if over-anxious, and especially if there seems to be some slight substance in what is being alleged, it is better by far to accept criticism at this stage as being honestly made and to offer some expression of sympathy and regret, without, perhaps, too much commitment.

\*       \*       \*

It pays to apologize. Nothing disarms a critic more completely or quickly than an admission of error, with or without a concession of fault. An apology evokes the sympathy of the recipient, himself in all probability a potent maker of mistakes. Like all generalizations, this is true only for the decent majority; there are others, weak themselves, who mistakenly see in an apology a sign of weakness and an invitation to be bolder in their criticism than they would otherwise have dared to be. There is nothing to be done with such people, except perhaps by those whose professional interest it is to study defects of personality.

Some find it hard to apologize. Their inability to do so may cause them to suffer a great deal more stress and trouble than they need. An early apology in a case which has given rise to a complaint, justified or not, may resolve the problem completely. In this connection I have often been struck by the curious analogy between a grievance in the mind and a malignant tumour. If a tumour is diagnosed early and treated, there is nowadays a very good chance of achieving a complete cure. If neglected, there is every possibility that the tumour will grow and invade surrounding tissues to the point of becoming inoperable. In addition, it will generate metastases far removed from the primary tumour. It is exactly so with grievances: if they are attended to early and in some degree remedied, there is every prospect that the complainant will feel relieved of resentment, turn away from contemplation of his grievance and get on with living a constructive life again.

But time and time again as Health Service Commissioner, I came across instances where a complaint had met first with an angry denial, followed by a series of argumentative exchanges by letter and embarrassing interviews, extending over many months. In some cases the grievance then became a matter of frank obsession, to the point where it dominated the complainant's whole life (and took up not a little of the life of the Health Service staff, too). Moreover, the complainant soon began to recall other grounds of grievance, only remotely connected with his original cause of complaint, in the sense that they may have arisen out of the same period of admission.

Convalescence

Soon, such people begin writing to more and more persons in higher and higher places in the attempt to justify the original initiative. In some the letter-writing, composition of articles for journals and statements for lawyers become a full-time and all-absorbing preoccupation.

I have the impression that reluctance to admit fault, or to apologize anyway, is rooted in some notion that this will always be construed in court or elsewhere as an admission of legal liability. For my own part, an immediate apology after some untoward event has no significance whatever. When I sat as a judge in civil matters, as I did at intervals over many years, it was sometimes suggested to a defendant by counsel that he had apologized because he knew himself to be in the wrong. I used to intervene to ask whether the next time counsel accidentally collided with someone in a crowded place and said: 'So sorry!', he would expect to pay damages for that unguarded exclamation. I hope that no judge worthy of the name would hold an apology to be evidence of an admission of liability unless the circumstances were such that the apology came in the course of a carefully considered response to a complaint and was made after due deliberation.[12]

\* \* \*

The phenomenon of dependency and its effect on the mind are now well established. Although these aspects of human behaviour are nowadays the subject of separate and scientific study, they are really both simple and obvious responses to the actions of others. If one submits to a regime in which even minor decisions, such as when to go to bed or when to get dressed, are taken for you; and if one is provided with clothing, food, and warmth without personal effort, it soon

12. For further consideration of this problem, see the Second Digression at page 46 below.

becomes easy, and then delightful, to accept the care and concern of others and to live in tranquil obedience. One may add to these powerful influences the awareness of having been rescued perhaps from disability or death by figures whom one sees daily performing these services for others and whose continuing presence is a reassurance. Finally, many patients may have experienced for the first time in their lives a period of being loved without stint simply for being in need of it and without being required to do anything in return. To abandon this sheltered existence even after quite a short experience of it requires an effort, which accounts for most of the complaints of premature discharge from hospital. It is of course an administrative necessity to consider whether and how the patient will manage during convalescence and what support there is for him at home. Failure to attend to this point may undo much of the good work which has been done in hospital.

It is a regrettable fact that time and again patients, and especially the elderly, are discharged from hospital without adequate administrative preparation. Often they are sent home to empty, cold, and locked premises, late in the evening, there to die very soon or to be readmitted to hospital next day. Frequently those who work in the community have not been warned of the patient's return and so cannot take steps which might alleviate these apparent inhumanities.

Fortunately most patients in reasonable general health have supportive families or relatives and are anxious to return home as soon as possible. For these no problem arises. But for the other group something more than a mere dismissal is called for. Some hospitals have a wonderful ability to make the discharge of a patient seem as important to them and as much a matter of concern as the original admission. Again it is the assurance of continuing interest and concern which raises routine health care to the level of excellence. It is that which further cements the relationship between the patient and those who have cared for him and means that when he is fully recovered he will probably put back into the service some of that care which has been expended upon him. This will take the form of fund-raising and similar activities which promote the interests of the hospital and those who work in it. Only a little thought is needed to perceive what is required to complete the successful treatment of a patient at this stage. There are some obviously unhappy turns of phrase, such as: 'We need your bed for someone else.' That may well be true and it is regrettably often said. But a more positive reason for sending the patient away is that he is fit to fend for himself and the final interview should be directed towards encouraging the patient to feel confident of this.

There are of course good clinical reasons for following up patients who have had a serious illness. But it may well be that the psychological benefits of the follow-up are even more important to the patient's perception of the care given to him. The natural sense of attachment and loyalty which the good patient feels to the hospital and its staff wherein and by whom he has been so well cared for, will make him anxious to return, to greet those whom he now regards as friends and to show them how well he has recovered. These visits, like other forms of health care, can be made occasions either of sterile and perfunctory routine or of mutual pleasure. Enormously long delays in dingy out-patient departments will make the patient feel that the hospital has lost interest in him. There are hospitals where the follow-up visit consists of a silent formal examination, perhaps the asking of the few essential questions and no more. Very soon appointments of that character are quietly abandoned by the patient and the relationship with the hospital dies with them. It should be possible both to keep the follow-up visit very short and yet to make it an occasion of renewal for friendship and mutual concern.

## THE SECOND DIGRESSION

It is a general principle of law in contracts of insurance that the insured shall not deliberately make his insurer liable. The purpose of a contract of insurance against mishaps such as legal liability to third parties for negligence is that the insurer is to be responsible for liability accidentally incurred, the probabilities of which he can calculate. Obviously, the insurer would not be willing to enter into an open-ended contract to insure someone against the consequences of deliberate acts. This principle is usually incorporated expressly into a contract of insurance by providing that the insured will not without the consent of the insurer make any admission of liability in respect of an incident insured against. Were it otherwise, the potential for fraud on the insurers is obvious.

There is little doubt that at any rate in years gone by, young doctors were indoctrinated with the notion that to admit liability for a mistake, or even to apologize, might jeopardize their right to indemnity under their contract of professional insurance. I know this belief still to be current and it may simply have been translated from motor or other insurance policies, where it is a condition of indemnity that admissions shall not be made without the insurers' prior consent.

In recent times the Medical Protection Society has openly declared that 'the defence societies make a substantial effort to encourage members to provide understandable explanations and to apologize when things may have gone wrong.'[13] Such a declaration is entirely admirable and what one would expect from the medical defence societies. But ringing declarations die away sooner than hoary old rumours and I am sure that the effect of the older and harsher dispensation persists.

This state of affairs is in no way the fault of the insurers. If

13. Letter to *British Medical Journal* 294:577 dated 28 February 1987 from Dr Ford of the Medical Protection Society.

there is fault at all, it is in the system. Insurance is a device for spreading the incidence of misfortune due to accident over a large part of the community, thus diminishing the impact of a mishap which might otherwise destroy an individual's life. Compulsory motor insurance ensures that there are large funds available at all times from which the victims of negligent accidents may be compensated. We are all anxious that these benevolent schemes shall be managed as economically as possible, because they add a cost to whatever activity is being insured against, which is disadvantageous to everyone.

It is therefore the duty of insurers to take care not to disburse the funds of the company without good cause. If they do so, the funds may be unnecessarily depleted and that can only result in an increase in premiums payable by all those insured. It is for this reason only that most insurance companies stipulate that no admissions should be made until they or experts on their behalf have had a reasonable chance to evaluate the incident which is likely to give rise to a claim and to decide whether liability should be contested or admitted. Thus viewed, the attitude of insurers is entirely reasonable. It is reassuring that the medical defence societies feel able to make an exception to the general rule in the particularly sensitive area of professional indemnity. I hope that the exception becomes more widely understood.

It remains true, or certainly did during my years as Health Service Commissioner, that some doctors and nurses felt obliged to adopt evasive and apparently unfeeling attitudes when patients or relatives asked about unexpectedly disappointing outcomes. Usually they would have liked to speak more frankly but felt inhibited from doing so.

Since this dilemma was a recurring feature of complaints which I received as Health Service Commissioner, I gave a good deal of thought to it over the years. The root of the problem is that apparent admissions of liability, whether oral or written, are admissible evidence on the issue of liability in subsequent legal proceedings. One solution to the problem might therefore be to create a new rule of evidence by which a consultation between doctor and patient or close relatives in the immediate aftermath of an unexpected and disappointing clinical outcome, should be inadmissible in subsequent proceedings. In legal terminology this would make such a consultation 'a privileged occasion', that is to say, the content of the consultation on both sides would be 'privileged' against subsequent production in evidence. In this way the dissatisfied patient or relative would not subsequently be able to take advantage in litigation of unguarded or over-generous concessions made in a consultation aimed at comfort and reassurance.

I believe that this expedient would go some way towards the relief of this persistent cause of complaint against the medical profession. But it would require legislation and the political difficulties are manifest. There are other professions to whom such a privilege might be attractive.

As a curious sidelight on this topic, I have often wondered how death-and-complications conferences have so long escaped the attentions of lawyers. According to legal theory, admissions of neglect made by one doctor to another on such occasions would by no means be privileged. Hearers of an admission of fault could be obliged to come to court and depose to what was said, however reluctantly. But the practicality of obtaining evidence in this way has no doubt deterred even claimants' lawyers from attempting it. For one thing, no one is obliged to make a written or oral statement prior to coming to court; it would be necessary therefore to call such a witness 'blind', that is to say, not knowing what his evidence might be, a practice so dangerous in advocacy that only the most foolish or desperate engage in it.

# 4
# The Patient's Relatives

'When the people complained,
it displeased the Lord.'
Numbers, xi, i.

Many a good clinician has observed that he has to treat the
relatives of the patient as well as the patient. Upright,
energetic, and noisy, they can indeed be more difficult to treat.
It is perhaps easy to underestimate the degree of their anxiety,
which may well exceed that of the patient himself. If he or she
is the breadwinner or housewife for a family, their future
without him or her may look bleak indeed. At some levels of
society it is usual to spend up to the limits of income each
week and to rely on the state to take care of emergencies. Even
in those families where savings and various forms of insurance
are usual, the loss even temporarily of the principal income
may be a serious business. For every dependent relative, the
illness of the provider creates an acute anxiety which probably
bites deeper, though unacknowledged, than the natural bonds
of love and affection. When relatives enquire after a beloved
patient, they are as much enquiring about their own future as
about the patient's, although they will not willingly admit it.

Talking to the relatives of the sick is laborious, exacting,
and time-consuming. It costs the service, whether national or
private, money. But it is as much the delivery of health care as
the prescribing of medication. In this, as in so many aspects of
human communication, listening is probably more important
than talking. A great deal of what relatives are anxious to say
will be clinically irrelevant. But to stem the flow of
recollection and foreboding is as damaging to the perception
of health care as it is ineffectual. It is ineffectual because every
interruption affords the opportunity for argument or further

49

elaboration of what has already been said. It is usually better in terms of both care and time to allow the flow to come to a natural halt from exhaustion of either the speaker or the material.

It requires very great patience and sympathy to stand in a corridor late at night after a long and hard day, listening to the outpouring of what may be needless or unjustified anxieties. Yet failure to do precisely that was in my experience a most prolific source of complaint. The ideal response in these circumstances is one so non-committal that the recipient will be quite unable later to recall what was said. Phrases such as: 'It's just anno domini, I'm afraid', or: 'He's had a good innings' are both remembered and resented. These are consolations only for those about to depart. By the living they are interpreted as admissions of defeat and at the same time as suggesting that the enquirer's anxiety is not justified by the circumstances of the patient. Neither of these implications is acceptable to a relative, however accurate they may be.

It is natural in the competent professional to feel confident in his diagnosis of some problem or in his decision as to how to treat it. That confidence, springing from a deep knowledge of the subject, can so easily develop into an intolerance of the possibility of being wrong. Just as firmness of purpose can develop into obstinacy, so can most virtues cross the invisible line beyond which they become vices.

Yet when one receives the bad news of a disaster to oneself or to someone very close, there is an instinctive reaching out for reassurance and confirmation as to even the most redoubtable opinion. This is an entirely natural and spontaneous reaction which should on no account be mistaken for a lack of respect for the opinion already received. It is indeed a weakness in any professional person to resent a request for a second opinion. The greater the confidence one has, the less is there to fear from a colleague's second opinion. And the more dire the opinion which has been given, the more should one feel glad to say, in effect, to a colleague: 'I think this is pretty straightforward, but just do me the favour of checking it out, would you?' It is a regrettable fact that each year the Health Service Commissioner receives some complaints in which it is clear that a request for a second opinion has been received with anger and resentment, to the shame and sorrow of some patient who sought only that further reassurance from expert people which helps them to bear a great blow.

Letters written to patients and relatives in response to anxious enquiries are equally important. In a far less important and dramatic context, I was much concerned when Parliamentary Commissioner for Administration and Health Service Commissioner, to ensure that the reports and letters which I wrote and signed should be as clear and unambiguous as it was possible to make them. I felt that both the citizen who paid me and the doctor, nurse, or civil servant whom I criticised deserved nothing less. I had also a selfish motive: I criticized with some severity whenever I came across it, that carelessness in the use of the written or spoken word which, as the failure of communication, I know to lie at the heart of the vast majority of complaints. I did not want to be guilty of the same lapse.

To cope with this problem, it was the invariable practice to arrange that anything important was read by more than one person before it left the office. If the subject-matter was one of unusual complexity or difficulty, it was best to ask someone who knew nothing of the topic to read the material and say whether he could easily understand it. I have sometimes wondered whether it might be both prudent and practicable for doctors when writing to lay people (or dare I say, to colleagues?), to have someone else on the hospital staff read through the letter or report and point out any obscurities or ambiguities. Letters to lay people could be read for this purpose by a friendly administrator. The point is that one always understands one's own writings without difficulty. The fallacious step is to assume that they will therefore be well understood by everyone else. When I read my own compositions, I comprehend them with the aid of a bank of factual and other data which has been used in the composition of the letter or report, but which is not available, or at any rate not in its entirety, to the reader. I therefore encounter no ambiguities when reading the material, or I resolve them instantly with the aid of my data-bank. Similarly, ellipses and inconsistencies are resolved almost without the necessity to think.

*       *       *

At the outset of this treatise I drew attention to the powerful inclination of human beings to blame some agency for misfortunes suffered. It seems unacceptable that a blind and unthinking fate should visit some fearful suffering on a wholly undeserving victim, without rhyme or reason. Perhaps such cruel and senseless affliction offends the rationality which is mankind's distinguishing attribute; and the more civilized a society is, the more eagerly does it seek for causes when disaster strikes, where primitive peoples would humbly blame themselves for failing to propitiate some malevolent deity.

Thus when an aircraft crashes, a ship capsizes, a nuclear power plant explodes, or some other catastrophe suddenly kills or injures our fellow-beings, we are disposed immediately to set up a more or less elaborate machinery of inquiry. The primary purpose of that inquiry will be to ascertain the facts of the happening: but the underlying thought throughout will be to discover whether any blame for its occurrence ought to be allocated to a person or persons responsible. There is nothing inherently malevolent or unreasonable in that thought, once it is conceded that man has some sort of control over the course of events which is being studied. For if the cause of the disaster can be traced to specific human error, the possibilities of preventing a recurrence are the greater.

It was in the spirit of detection and prevention of the causes of disaster that many lawsuits alleging medical negligence were formerly brought. There was also another reason: many complainants writing to the Health Service Commissioner asserted quite convincingly that they neither wanted nor needed money but were determined to get explanations which were denied to them outside court proceedings, for the reasons to which I referred in Chapter 3.

Many doctors are known to detest legal proceedings and the lawyers who conduct them. It must admittedly be a very unpleasant ordeal to be closely questioned by a layman about one's exercise of a professional judgment which may be as much a matter of art as of technical knowledge. The negative aspect of the judicial process is that the questions may be very hard to answer and thus give the spectators at a public inquiry an impression of medical competence which is unfairly inaccurate and misleading. The positive aspect is that submission to close questioning by intelligent laymen brings one to a clearer vision of one's true knowledge and motivation as opposed to one's speculative or intuitive assumptions and resistance to change.

I once had the privilege of knowing an orthopaedic surgeon of great eminence. He frequently accepted invitations to give expert evidence in court proceedings. This surprised many of his lesser colleagues who spoke of their heavy commitments, huge operating lists, and distaste for having to explain elementary medical propositions to ignorant, glib, and superficial cross-examiners. This was not the view of matters expressed to me by my friend. He said that there was no process he knew of which brought him to a clearer understanding of what his work was about, of the validity of his basic assumptions, of the accuracy of his diagnoses and prognoses, than the formal and public examination of those matters in court.

Several consequences, all good, flowed from this positive attitude to the giving of evidence. The reports prepared by my friend were of a luminous clarity which ended by making them acceptable to both sides in a dispute, so that he actually entered the witness-box less and less often. Secondly, if he did go into the box, it was virtually impossible to cross-examine him. This was because he had so carefully and honestly searched his mind for what he really knew about the matter under review and could honestly and unequivocally assert, that attempts to show illogicality or inconsistency were bound to fail. Indeed, attempts to undermine his evidence resulted only in his re-stating his propositions in yet clearer terms, thus producing the opposite to the desired effect of cross-examination. Only incompetent counsel persisted after the first few questions, thus doing their client's case unlimited damage. My friend had also both the eminence and the modesty to be able to say: 'I simply do not know the answer to that question and I do not believe that anyone else does', a non-answer which could not of course be cross-examined, but which greatly strengthened his evidence on those matters wherein he declared an opinion.

It follows from the tenor of my previous observations that the judicial process can be cruelly revelatory of undisciplined mental processes in medical as in other professional fields. But surely this is as it should be. In an age much given to doubt and suspicion of competence and motivation (especially those of others) rigorous self-examination is necessary for survival. The searching, magnifying, revealing eye of the television camera ruthlessly exposes the weaving, shifting, hesitating, prevaricating subject of its unblinking gaze. It is as well to be prepared for an encounter which may come the way of any doctor of some distinction in his field and who may need publicly to declare and vindicate his decisions, his opinions, or his researches.

One should not therefore be scornful of the legal process for resolving disputes, even in such delicate and difficult matters as actions for medical negligence. That said, however, it must regrettably be noted that more such actions are being brought nowadays than used to be the case and that it is difficult to avoid the impression that many of the claimants are actuated more by greed or revenge than by any constructive motive.

The worst excesses in this direction seem to have been suffered in North America, where the so-called 'contingency fee'[14] must be largely to blame. The evil propensities of this pernicious arrangement are manifold. An honest lawyer who accepts a case on a fee-contingent basis out of charity may go without proper reward for much skilful and arduous toil. A dishonest lawyer who knows he must win his case if he is to be paid, is tempted to search for dishonest witnesses and to rehearse even honest witnesses in what they must say in court. These odious practices occur quite commonly but never in this country.

A further evil consequence is that courts, (and especially those where juries try civil claims) are apt to inflate the damages to take account of the fact that a large part of any sum they award to a claimant will go straight to the lawyers. This inflationary factor has to be provided for by the professional indemnity insurers, who increase insurance premiums, as they must, to cover the actual claims experience. The burden of the premiums inevitably finds its way on to the shoulders of the public in terms of increased medical charges.

For the practitioner in such conditions, the inhibitory effects are well enough known. They include a reluctance to give even first aid to the victims of accident, fear of innovation or clinical enterprise, and the needless deployment of diagnostic procedures and aids.

By contrast, the British lawyer has always demanded a fee even for reading and preparing a case which is subsequently settled. He receives his full fee for a case which goes to trial even if he loses after many weeks of struggle. So although it is more agreeable to win than to lose, it is not at all a matter of

14. A 'contingency fee' is one the payment of which is contingent on a successful outcome to the lawsuit. The fee is commonly a substantial percentage of any damages recovered. If the suit fails, the lawyer gets nothing.

survival. There is therefore no incentive to stoop to the kind of deplorable impropriety which I mentioned earlier.

It is very much to be hoped that the disease of persistent litigation, so prevalent in the United States, will not spread to this country, although there have been recent signs of an increase, according to the professional indemnity societies. The media made much of the first £1m award of damages for medical negligence in this country, just as irresponsibly as they invariably describe pay rises in gross rather than net terms. In fact the courts do no more than express in less valuable currency the same costs of disability which have been heads of damages for very many years.

For the disappointed patient or relative, the lawsuit is the ultimate and most damaging catharsis of complaint, leaving both sides exhausted and unhappy.

One often hears propounded the idea of a legal system under which there would be 'strict liability for the victims of medical accidents'. Thus vaguely stated, with all the imprecision of a notion which has not been properly considered, such an arrangement has a superficial appeal. It is necessary to consider first, what exactly a system of strict liability would mean, and secondly what it would imply.

'Strict liability' in practical terms must mean a liability on someone to pay damages in money (no other remedy being envisaged) without there being any fault on the part of the person paying. In those countries which have introduced such a scheme, a government department or body is in effect substituted for all those persons who might otherwise have been involved in what might be described as a 'medical accident'. The department will decide when a decline in health following or in the course of treatment amounts to an accident. That may be a finely judged thing. Is a cardiac arrest due to vagal inhibition at first incision an accident? Nothing has gone wrong with the operation thus far. Presumably those who in the prime of life are stricken by multiple sclerosis have not had 'accidents', although the effect on the sufferers may be as sudden and devastating as if they had. Do we have less compassion for them or any less desire to see them compensated so far as may be for a life of increasing disability and suffering?

The truth is that definition of the expression 'accidental injury' is far from easy and has already occupied many volumes of law reports. The time-honoured phraseology of insurance law, which defines an accident as caused by 'external, violent and visible means', would hardly serve for an accidental over-exposure to radiation which might often fail to comply with any of those three adjectival qualifications and never with the last two.

The concept of strict liability therefore runs at the outset into difficulties of definition and identification which the idea of fault does not. Fault requires an identifiable act or omission of something which either should not have been done or was wrongly neglected, the doing or not doing of which was a cause of the injury.

Having thus narrowed the field of liability to identifiable acts or omissions, it is usually not too difficult to find the doer or omitter who is the person to be made liable.

But that is by no means the end of the matter. 'Fault' and 'liability for fault' go naturally hand-in-hand in the estimation of right-thinking people. 'No liability without fault' has as righteous a ring as 'No taxation without representation'. This is no lawyer's subtlety: '. . . disgraceful, it is—he (or they) ought to be made to pay' is the language of the man or woman 'on the Clapham omnibus'. It comes naturally to think that those who hurt others by their fault should make good the damage, just as it seems unjust that an innocent person should have to pay for injuries caused through no fault of his. This is because both 'fault' and 'liability' have fundamental moral connotations; remove them and you remove the moral basis for this part of our civil law. I suggest that this could not but have a damaging influence eventually on the relationship between doctor or nurse and patient. As I pointed out in an early chapter, there is a strong moral basis of surrender and committal for this relationship. If it were to become the law that neither the giving of one's best care to a patient nor the withholding of it had any relevance to the question of liability if anything went wrong, can it be doubted that the relationship would be damaged? In the broader field of human activities, for example the driving of motor vehicles, I suggest that strict liability would be a disastrous innovation.

One hopes it would be less so in the field of medicine, where the majority of practitioners give of their best in any event. But it is not to be expected that any profession would be uninfluenced by the reflection that, do or neglect what they might, they were going to be liable anyway if anything went wrong and nothing short of murder or manslaughter would affect the outcome. Always accompanying fault is the stigma of blame. It is felt as a disgrace, at any rate to an extent varying with the degree of fault, to be held to blame for someone else's sufferings. The fear of being held to blame is a stimulus to us all to do our best and it is one which all but the most saintly of us need in the repetitive toil of exercising our professional or other skills.

Then there are serious practical implications. A system of law under which liability is based on fault holds that the person at fault is a wrongdoer. He should therefore be made to compensate his victim fully in so far as money can do that. Awards of damages thus include loss of earning capacity for the future, past and continuing expenses incurred by reason of the injuries caused, and a notional sum for past and future pain and suffering. For a young claimant the total of these sums may be a formidable amount. If every victim of a medical mishap were to be entitled to compensation without proof of fault, the cost to the state seems likely to be an annual sum so great that the majority of people would say that we could not afford such generosity.

New Zealand, which has a system of liability without fault for accidental injury, has been obliged to limit drastically the compensation obtainable under the scheme, in order to be able to afford it. There they have eliminated from the assessment some of the heads of damage which we regard as essential to fair compensation. Non-earners may get nothing at all under the scheme. Those who extol the arrangements in other countries and criticize ours do not always draw attention to these important differences.

Nor would litigation be eliminated altogether by such a scheme. Although proof of fault causing the injuries alleged would no longer be an issue in court proceedings, there would without doubt be arguments about whether the injuries to be compensated were in fact caused by the relevant accident and as to the amount of compensation to be awarded if they were.

A Royal Commission on Civil Liability and compensation for Personal Injury[15] concluded in March 1978 that a 'no-fault scheme' was inappropriate in the field of medicine, except for the special case of volunteers in a clinical trial. The Commission did recommend a no-fault scheme for injuries suffered in road traffic accidents, to be financed by a tax on petrol. Despite the great distinction of the members of the Commission, one may respectfully take leave to doubt the wisdom of the latter idea and in the nine years since their report, there has been no move to implement their recommendation. The special case of volunteers in clinical trials has been provided for voluntarily by the pharmaceutical industry and local ethics committees in the National Health Service.

Plainly I lack both the space and the competence to deal with this difficult topic at length. The Royal Commission treated it exhaustively and with much applied learning, in addition to visiting countries where such schemes were to be found to judge their effectiveness. Their report may be warmly recommended to interested readers.

15. 1977–78 Cmnd 7054 I–III.

# 5
# Epilogue

'... 'tis true that a good play needs no epilogue.'
*A.Y.L.* Epil. 3

In a normal year a healthy working man or woman may pay up to £1,590 per annum towards health insurance and pay it compulsorily by deduction from earnings at source. Under the national health scheme, therefore, health care is free only at the time of delivery. The patient's contribution to the care received is not negligible and a healthy person may have paid a very substantial part of the cost of the service actually delivered to him or her by the time some illness requires hospital treatment.

Because a bill is not rendered and a cheque received at the time of discharge, some doctors have come to feel that patients are the recipients of charity or a 'welfare hand-out' for which they should be humbly grateful. And because a modern doctor possesses and displays a great armoury of technical knowledge, while his patient lies inert and silent, some doctors have come to think that they are somehow superior beings. The fault can hardly be described as prevalent, but if it has any general currency, it tends to be among doctors young and old who lack the imagination to envisage their patients as they normally are when in good health, possessed perhaps of a range of knowledge and skills at least the equal of those of the medical profession. Such practitioners are apt to treat their patients in a manner which is at best patronizing and at worst arrogant.

How this has come about I cannot tell. Without doubt there are great numbers of doctors at the top of their profession whose breadth of vision and knowledge of other than medical disciplines make it impossible for them to behave as I have just described. I throw out for consideration the possibility, which I have discussed with undergraduates in other faculties, that medical students are apt to remain together overmuch as a group during their long and demanding years of medical education. The fearful slog of recapitulating medical learning to the point we have now reached absorbs all the time and energy of serious medical students. Perhaps they see others finding time and energy to pursue all manner of extraneous activities and so come to regard other disciplines as superficial. A man holding a doctorate in a biological science whose work at a university brought him into collaboration with doctors, recently told me that he had decided to acquire a medical qualification. He had taken this step because it was the only way in which he could avoid the irritation of being constantly looked down upon by medically qualified colleagues.

Such attitudes go hand-in-hand with resentment of criticism. A patient's complaint often seems to carry a critical implication. Doctors will readily recall the purely medical and Greek derivation of the word 'critic', one who was well able to judge the point in the progress of a disease when an important development or change takes place. Only by long usage, or misusage, has 'critical' come to have the secondary meaning of adverse judgment. Every rational complaint contains the germ of a judgment on a crucial point, if one takes the trouble to discern it and to that extent only is it truly critical. That critical element in complaints is well worth attending to because it may give a clear lead to the delivery of better medical care. The difficulty is to divest the complaint of its prickly husk of emotion, animosity, and resentment, leaving only the useful kernel from which good practices may grow. More easily said than done, perhaps, but much is learned from the disasters and ensuing complaints which have overtaken others. It is, for example, no longer possible to interchange oxygen and nitrous oxide lines in operating theatres.

Accepting complaints and criticism about oneself is hard, there is no denying it. Reading complaints and criticism about others is a great deal easier and perhaps one learns more readily that way. I spoke earlier of my dislike of proverbs and catch-phrases and another one of pernicious import is: 'There, but for the grace of God, go I'. The proper reaction to learning of someone else's downfall is: 'While in possession of my reason, there is no possibility that I would have gone that way and with the help of God and my colleagues I am not going that way in the future either'. Nor should the study of complaints be regarded solely as a backward-looking and therefore negative activity, any more than is the post mortem examination of a body, from which so much may be learned which is of use to the living.

So I end as I began. The patient suffers from a complaint of which, if it progresses, he complains. If he is not treated kindly and considerately he may complain of that, too, quite apart from the treatment of his illness of which he may also complain. All of this complaining is part of the course of illness, some of which is justified by observable causes and some of which is not. But in any event it has to be dealt with as part of the medical commitment, with such patience and forbearance as a good doctor can command. And even when a particular patient oversteps the limits of those virtues, it is well to look back a little and wonder what went wrong and whether in some way a similar disagreeable experience might be avoided in the future.

As for the patient—well, he is in a dilemma. He may love in the truest sense the doctors and nurses who have cared for him in his extremity. At the same time he may have perceived in the course of his illness a number of ways in which their care could have been delivered so much better. He may be saddened at the realization that so much that was good in the service was marred by some failure so easy to rectify. He may say to himself, if he has a healthy and rational mind, 'Well, what is it to me? I am safely home, restored to my loved ones and fully recovered. It seems ungrateful to moan about it'. So he says nothing. If in an access of public spirit, he decides to

*Epilogue*

write a letter about the defects he saw, he may sadden those who cared for him, sour a happy human relationship and even get himself and his family marked down as potential troublemakers. It has happened. This is the patient's dilemma.

63